Healthy and Delighted: How to Get in Shape and Live a Better Life

By

Rebecca Cora

Healthy and Delighted:

How to Get in Shape and Live a Better Life

Healthy and Delighted:

How to Get in Shape and Live a Better Life

TABLE OF CONTENT

Introduction

Every day, we keep ourselves preoccupied with what is most important to us. Often, just making a living and surviving is sufficient. By doing this, we occasionally ignore or forget about the extra things that are required to maintain a healthy balance in our lives. They are even more important in providing true meaning to our world. Your health must be taken seriously.

Exercise, a low-fat, high-fiber diet, and a desire to do so are the keys to good health. Naturally, you'll also need to stop engaging in bad behaviors like smoking, binge drinking, or abusing drugs, including prescription medications.

There isn't a miracle pill that will cause you to lose weight without making an effort. There is no specific diet that enables you to eat a lot of food and lose weight quickly. No ab-machine or exercise bike that you catch on an infomercial in the middle of the night is going to change your life.

I suppose we all know the key to losing weight. Eat healthily, move more, and maintain a happy outlook. Yes, we're all aware of it.

But if you've ever struggled with your weight, you know it's not always that simple. Eating healthfully is challenging when you're constantly hungry, everything that's good for you tastes bad, and you're moving at the top pace. Fast food is very alluring when you have a full day planned out from the moment you wake up until you go to bed at night. Exercise is time-consuming, challenging, and even downright awful! That positive outlook, though, is rather simple. After you get beyond the hunger pangs and the sore muscles, you'll notice that you haven't eaten anything you've enjoyed in a week and a half and that the bike seat has left you with blisters in awkward places.

After that, maintaining a good attitude is simple. No, I suppose it isn't.
Exercise is the key to excellent health, as is a low-fat, high-fiber diet.

Those who take care of their bodies tend to be in good health. You will experience more benefits in many different ways when you improve your health now. You'll find yourself doing things you've never done before you realize it.

Even though our earthly lives are merely in the greater power's control, we may still make an effort to have happy and healthy lives. We will live longer if we take care of our bodies and have complementary lifestyles.

Would you like to be happy, healthier, and live longer? Reading this e-Book can assist you in achieving your objectives if you want.

Chapter 1:
The Fundamentals

The following are some things to think about to get you started with the fundamentals.

- Rest will improve your physical health and reduce your tension and anxiety.

You can think more clearly after sleeping. Establish a good sleeping schedule. Find out how much sleep you require. Take a 30-minute sleep if you aren't working throughout the day; it might make you feel better at night. You'll have to determine how much sleep your body needs because everyone's bodies are different.

- The appropriate food, vitamins, and nutrition will enable you to lead the life you desire.

The body requires nourishment to function, therefore if we don't eat right, we'll be starving our essential organs and they won't work properly. Additionally bad for the body and making the heart work harder is gluttony.

The reality that we are spiritual beings in addition to physical beings is overlooked by the adage "eat less and move more."

But something needs to be done. The rate at which people are gaining weight is worrying. From the oldest to the youngest among us, we are gaining weight at rates never before witnessed.

Some doctors and other medical professionals assert that consuming wholesome foods is more important than exercising. But is it true?

- Daily exercise will increase the likelihood that you won't have brittle bones and tight joints as you age.

Your pulse will improve with exercise, ensuring a healthier lifestyle and keeping you from feeling lethargic. With exercise, stress, and anxiety may be reduced. If you're not exercising, start right away. Don't start with intense workouts. Easy leg lifts, arm lifts, and stretching are all OK. If you can use stairs, move slowly up and down them several times every day. You can gradually increase the amount of exercise you give your body after a week. Give it some time.

- If we want to achieve long-term weight loss, we must focus on the psychological, emotional, and physiological aspects.

This journey will be as challenging and unpleasant as following the toughest diet. Although it could be, it isn't. You may increase your willpower, metabolic rate, and positive thoughts about reducing weight by employing a few straightforward tactics. Additionally, you can get rid of hunger pangs and anxiety related to your current weight.

Don't worry if you haven't tried anything like this before because you can do it yourself or get a friend or professional to help you with it.

Here are a few simple methods you can use to help with weight loss. Despite being straightforward, they are incredibly effective. Even while you still need to diet and exercise, using these techniques will make it simpler.

Start by relaxing and clearing your mind. Just take a time to unwind, let go of any worries, and put everything else aside.

Think in your mind that you're already slim. I know that this feels unusual, but if you wish to lose weight it helps to convince yourself that it's possible. If your brain rebels and tries to tell you something different, simply replace the thought with the ide.a you're thin and healthy and don't fret about it. It will take some time to train your subconscious to be thin. Spend a few moments just "knowing" you're slim and trim. You don't even have to picture it. In fact, it is more beneficial to your deeper self if you do not visualize it.

Now imagine your day. "See" yourself consuming a healthy breakfast. Do what you need to till lunch. Imagine the time passing without you feeling particularly hungry, and imagine sitting down to a lunch of nutritious items that you prepared earlier.

Recognize that mistakes will happen, but you'll let them slide. Is it difficult to see yourself exercising and loving it? Of course, but nothing too difficult for you! In the same manner, hurry through dinner.

You'll notice that you don't have a particularly sweet tooth, nor do you feel hungry. Will you take a quick snack before going to bed?

You have the choice.

It's important to use conceptual thought as much as you can in this situation. Do your best if you haven't mastered the art of thinking in concepts yet.

- Your body will be able to get rid of toxins, bacteria, and other things it doesn't need with the help of water.

Only water will effectively clean out your system. It is strongly advised that you have enough water each day.

The next time you need to buy anything to drink, keep this in mind and buy a bottle of water. Without the sugar and other components in soda pop, you'll save money and improve your health.

- Stop yourself from becoming hurt.

Do you enjoy riding a bike? Put a helmet on. Avoid saying, "That's not for me." Every day, bicycle accidents injure both children and adults. Keep your head and brain safe.

- Use effective lotions and moisturizers to shield the skin from excessive sun exposure.

Moisturizers and lotions will assist maintain healthy skin. The skin will begin to shrink and break down as we age. Using high-quality lotions and moisturizers will assist your body in maintaining healthy skin.

- An individual needs to reduce the stress, despair, and tension in their life.

It stresses the heart in addition to being bad for your emotional condition. These things need to be under control, and we need to learn to relax.

- You must stop smoking.

Not much else to add about that. It tastes bad, smells bad, and isn't good. It's not fun for your heart or lungs either. Let it go.

- Keep an eye on the doctor's appointments.

Visit your doctor as often as they would like you to. Get checked out annually to make sure everything is fine with you.

We must launch a campaign for preventive care.

Chapter 2:
The Detailed Ideas

Reaching within and relying on your instincts will help you find happiness. You must adopt a healthy lifestyle free of drugs, chemicals, substances, special habits, behavior, and so on if you want to live longer and be healthier. To improve your metabolism, bones, joints, and muscles, you must exercise.

Next, we'll examine several distinct ideas in succession. Keep in mind that they will be creating strong spiritual fields around you, so be sure to keep your ideas and conceptions as steady and as clear as you possibly can.

Greater Depth

Humans need spiritual, mental, and physical nourishment to stay healthy and powerful. Prayer, a deeper understanding of the teachings from the higher power, and continual mental and physical hygiene are all examples of spiritual nutrition. The body is our temple, and if we use drugs, eat unhealthy food, drink too much alcohol, or participate in harmful behavior, we'll endure misery, poor health, and a shorter lifespan.

Some of the things we do in life could be harmful to us. Without adequate sleep, we may eventually develop heart problems as well as other health issues. To live a healthier life, you must break negative habits and adopt new healthy habits. Most people don't realize that the way they act could be adding to their stress and distress.

Each health plan should start with the right combination of exercise, a healthy diet, and rest. You may lead a healthier life if you stay with a healthy diet and take the right vitamins and supplements. The fact that unhealthy additives are added to our food, which affects the lives of millions of people, is one of the major problems of today.

Things that are added to foods, which lead to weight gain and desires, are one of the reasons why obesity is on the rise.

Many people only pay attention to what they want to hear and ignore what they want to ignore. We occasionally need to consider the facts. If your friends or loved ones confide in you that you're drinking too much, pay attention to what they have to say because you're not only harming yourself but also others you care about.

An individual may feel distressed if an emotional reaction has a negative outcome. An individual's life expectancy and level of wellness are both decreased by distress.

Rephrasing sentences could improve communication with others. If inactive listening occurs, relationships frequently end. For instance, when someone is upset, they could attack them emotionally, which causes the other person to respond adversely. All of this results in depression and will subsequently reduce your life through illness.

We all occasionally daydream or take a brief break, but if we go too far and use it as a means of avoiding reality, we only end up harming ourselves. You must control this type of behavior and/or habit if you want to be happier.

Judging is a different significant issue. Numerous people pass judgment, but very rarely do they genuinely come to know the subject of their judgment. Stop passing judgment on other people if you want to be happier. Stop criticizing people if you don't want to be criticized yourself. Remember: Treat people fairly as you would like to be treated.

There are options for good and negative. You'll almost certainly find something positive about someone if you're looking for it. You'll probably find someone's flaws if you're looking for them. Your decision is yours.

Unfortunately, it does occasionally happen for the bad to take control of people's life and crush the good within them.

Many believe they can read minds. Instead of listening to what is stated to them, they frequently misquote others. Avoid doing it. The following are specific exercises to perform for a healthier and leaner body:

Keep the idea of energy with you at all times. As energy flows through you, feel it. thrilling and buzzing through your system. Your metabolic rate will increase as a result. Feel it throughout your entire body. Keep holding for at least one minute.

Keep the idea of warmth in mind. Warming up every area of your being after starting in the center. Your metabolism will increase as a result. Maintain once more for at least a minute.

Carry the notion of not being hungry. You must be careful not to completely rob oneself of appetite because this is so potent. In actuality, this will lessen your bodily desire and appetite. Keep going like this for a minute.

Hold onto the idea of bliss at last. No matter if you desire to reduce weight, everyone should do this! Your confidence will be raised to the point that you can maintain your workout and nutrition plan.

Many extra things may be done to assist someone in losing weight through spiritual practices. Exercise, for instance, might be more enjoyable if pain management strategies are used, as well as basic mood-lifting techniques.

With a little assistance, you may change your internal and outward perceptions of the kind of foods that are tasty. Increased metabolism may cause the body to eliminate fat rather than store it.

Of course, you'll need to keep an eye on your diet.

Yes, exercise is good for you and should be a regular component of your routine. However, using these and other spiritual healing methods may make losing weight easier and more effective while also improving your quality of life.

Try to recruit a friend to help you if you want to try these tactics but are concerned that you lack the necessary skill set.

If you can't do that, you can attempt to hire an expert to help you in the short run. However, with enough practice, you can learn to accomplish all of these things on your own. You can influence these circumstances.

The decision is now yours: will you take control of your weight or will you carry on as usual?

You have the choice

Chapter 3:
Be Kinder To Yourself

Everybody has days when it feels like the weight of the world is on their shoulders. We could feel that living a healthier, longer, and happier life is unattainable at this moment. Some of us can handle strain as it comes our way, but others find it difficult.

To lead a happier life, one must change certain behaviors, ways of thinking, routines, and other aspects of one's behavior.

Your health will suffer if you allow bad actions to rule your mind.

Better Methods of Living

When you paraphrase during a conversation, you are summarizing. Reiterating information clarifies communication, which fosters the growth of a much richer relationship. Let's look at an example to help you understand how paraphrasing can lessen conflict, ease tension, improve health, and prevent stress eating.

Sue: John, I have to go dress shopping for the approaching occasion.

You want a new dress, John?

Sue: I really would like a new dress.

John: You say you want to get a new dress for the next occasion. So, are you requesting my approval to purchase the dress? (Clarifying)

Sue: Yes, my dear.

John: That's okay with me. Purchase a new dress if you desire one.

Sue Thanks.

Even though this paraphrasing is straightforward, it is evident how it clarifies the dialogue. Passive listening will be stopped by paraphrasing. Additionally, it will correct any accusations, presumptions, or misinterpreted communications. You both benefit from paraphrasing because you both feel heard and taken note of. Communication is two-way, and by paraphrasing, you can control irate feelings, which typically get stronger when information is misunderstood. Additionally, it's an excellent technique to improve memory. When emotions are turbulent, they have an impact on the heart, which frequently results in poor health. You must have emotional self-control if you want to live a happier life. Clarifying helps you control your feelings.

Negativity simply causes health problems and relationship problems. It causes melancholy and negative thoughts. Negative energy (emotions) is essentially self-denial. It's a serious issue that has people suffering. Damaged energy (emotional reaction) can have a variety of negative effects, including heart failure, hypertension, strokes, and other health issues.

Positive energy will often reflect on others, and it will frequently transmit warmth. If you can develop good energy, you'll shine like a star and it will make you happy within.

What's the problem? We all deal with tension daily.

Stress cannot be avoided. Your life might become easier if you learn how to reduce pressures and tension.

Engaging in stretching exercises is one of the finest strategies to reduce stress. In light of this, we can offer some advice on how to lessen stress. Regular exercise helps you improve your energy levels, sleep quality, self-respect, and other aspects of your life.

Today, stress is one of the main causes of death worldwide.

Tension is the primary trigger for many illnesses. The initial action you. The indications of strain must be recognized. You might be able to fight back and win the battle if you can spot the warning signs. You're probably anxious

if you feel tense, jittery, or restless is taking over. Tension is indicated by sensitivity, negative thinking, and taking offense at what others say to you. You may be experiencing tension if you are jerking uncontrollably, biting your nails, pulling your hair, or wriggling your knees. Tension might be indicated by nausea, irregular bowel movements, diarrhea, frequent smoking, and a dependency on alcohol or narcotics. If you start to get irritable all the time and have little patience, you're under stress. Frequently, irritation develops into tension, stress, and aggressive or compulsive actions.

Stress is likely the cause of your frequent forgetfulness, difficulty focusing, mental fatigue, detached feeling, and inability to think clearly. Signs include feeling very worn out and pressured. Low self-esteem, anxiety, panic attacks, rage, bitterness, crying for nothing, moodiness, nightmares, and the inability to express joy are some possible symptoms.

Stress can cause your muscles to tense up and make you feel exhausted. Back, head, shoulder, and neck pain are likely to occur. You can have eye fatigue and twitching, especially in the area around the corners of your eyes. Frequently, the mouth feels dry and the jaw feels stiff. The hands' palms could feel. The fingertips will feel cold and perspiration-filled. You can regularly have stomach, bladder, and urine issues, as well as heartburn.

Additionally, you can encounter heart palpitations, weight gain or loss, headaches, colds, hyperventilation, and other symptoms.

Knowing the foundations of eating a balanced diet is one method to reduce stress. Stress management is essential. Eating three balanced meals or five little amounts of food each day is essential. Avoid eating fast when you are eating; instead, take your time and allow the meal to fully digest. Incorporate 5 servings of fruits and vegetables each day.

You can find it beneficial to have a glass of water half an hour before and after meals.

Regular exercise will improve your mood, sleep quality, energy level, self-esteem, and self-assurance. You'll feel and look fantastic. A typical schedule should include daily tasks that take 20 to 30 minutes. If you have trouble getting moving, start slowly and build up to a complete workout.

The position is important. Always examine your posture before working out; it should be aligned. Keeping it straight may prevent bone-related illnesses and promote improved breathing, which eases stress. You'll feel more at ease, have more self-assurance, and look younger, fitter, and leaner as a result of it. Additionally, it will increase energy and vigor, which is essential.

Attempt to go to bed at the same time every night. Tension will decrease throughout sleep. If you have trouble falling asleep, consider changing your bedroom. You might feel better after a change. When you're trying to fall asleep, keep the room quiet and dark. Make sure your mattress and pillow support your posture and give you a comfortable feeling. Avoid using coffee, smoking, or drinking before going to bed. You can exercise an hour before bed to make yourself tired. Get out of bed and read a book if you frequently wake up during the night and find it difficult to fall back asleep.

Teach your brain to relax and think positively just when you are awake. Try to concentrate on one task at a time to promote relaxation and memory. Try not to worry; instead, take action.

Your attitude is extremely important. A positive view or attitude motivates you to carry out your plans and ambitions.

Proper breathing is necessary for both stretching activities and meditation.

Breathe normally while working out, doing meditation, etc. Become conscious of your breathing and work on doing it correctly. This will put you at ease.

Stretching may aid in flexing the joints, which supports strong muscles. By stretching, you'll clear your airways and feel more at ease.

You might want to utilize meditation before starting an exercise program. Positive thinking can be implemented and your mind can be cleared through meditation. Yours has to work on focusing your attention during meditation. While some prefer to focus on objects, others prefer to listen to subtle sounds. Enlightenment of the spiritual consciousness is what meditation is. The right way to meditate involves maintaining good posture, breathing, centering, and attitude. The practice of meditation will encourage awareness and calmness. Health, longevity, and happiness are all increased when the mind and body are relaxed.

Chapter 4:
Our Mentality and Supplements

We can exercise and try to eat foods that won't infect our bodies as much as possible. To live longer and better lives, we must make decisions. By growing our fruits and vegetables, we may avoid using dangerous chemicals that could taint natural vitamins. We might wish to use supplements even more.

Purchasing

Scientific advancements have made it possible to live longer and in better health, since they have greatly increased life expectancy and decreased the likelihood of developing age-related illnesses. Science is currently making great efforts to uncover solutions to live healthier lives while delaying aging because the circumstances frequently result in serious health issues and ultimately death.

What can I individually do to prolong my life?

Exercise, maintain a healthy diet, and understand supplements. keep seeing your doctor and ask for guidance. Take action and the time to listen.

Let's examine a few supplements. REMEMBER TO ALWAYS CHECK WITH YOUR DOCTOR FIRST!

The pituitary gland releases the hormone known as HGH (Human Growth Hormone). In medicine, HGH is used to treat adult growth hormone deficiency as well as pediatric growth problems. Reduced body fat, increased muscle mass, bone density, and energy levels are only a few of the reported effects on GH-deficient patients (but not on healthy people). Other reported effects to include improved immune system performance and skin tone/texture.

Growth hormone replacement therapy has gained popularity recently in the battle against aging and obesity.

Our bodies include raging hormones, which stop manufacturing or secreting appropriate substances that promote better living. Dehydroepiandrosterone (DHEA)-

containing products boost the immune system, aiding in illness prevention.

Long-term DHEA supplementation has been found in a few small, randomized clinical studies to improve mood, treat depression, or reduce insulin resistance. It is known that regular exercise improves the body's ability to produce DHEA. Some claim that the increase in endogenous DHEA brought on by calorie restriction contributes to the extended life expectancy that is known to be connected to calorie restriction.

Ginkgo has been shown to slow down the aging process while speeding up health problems. It is a plant extract that encourages consciousness and healthier brain function. In Germany, doctors use ginkgo products to treat patients with dementia, poor blood circulation, and other conditions. By providing natural nutrients, the product helps to improve brain cells.

Studies are being conducted to demonstrate whether ginkgo may improve memory in people with Alzheimer's disease. Recent research has shown that persons with Alzheimer's disease show symptoms of remembering and interacting with others more successfully than people who take other natural herbs. Additionally, many dealing with PTSD and MPD have found relief from this herbal extract. The only hazards of using ginkgo are those associated with the consumption of herb that contains warfarin, coumadin, aspirin, ginger, aspirin, aspirin, or feverfew.

A polyunsaturated vegetable oil called flax-seed oil contains nutrients including omega-3 fatty acids and other fatty acids. Omega-3 has shown promise in lowering blood pressure, cholesterol, triglycerides, and sticky platelets, among other things.

The natural fats found in our bodies' tissues are called triglycerides. The use of flax seed oils may reduce the number of heart attacks and strokes. High-dense lipoproteins (HDLS), the good cholesterol that protects the heart by slowing artery occlusion, were also discovered to benefit from omega-3. As a result, Omega-3 removes LDL from the bloodstream to facilitate flow.

It has been demonstrated that flaxseed oil can reduce or stop the growth of breast cancers. Lignin is a substance that prevents or treats cancer. A substance based on estrogen is lignin.

Using flaxseed oils also helps to alleviate chronic cardiac diseases.

Written reports claim that the sole risk is that you might put on weight. Due to their high-calorie content, flaxseed oils must be a part of your daily caloric intake if you want to reduce your risk of weight gain.

A hormone called melatonin is released by our pineal glands. It has a positive impact on mood and nerves. Studies suggest that melatonin augmentation may slow dementia and Alzheimer's. Additionally, it has been shown to slow cancer growth, tumor growth, and the aging process.

Stress can cause low levels of melatonin, which can lead to anxiety, panic attacks, continual concern, trauma, and other symptoms like these. The drawback is that as we age, our bodies stop producing melatonin properly.

Melatonin pills may be able to ease your nervousness and help you get a restful night's sleep if you struggle with anxiety and sleeping problems.

You'll feel better every day if you can get enough restorative sleep and relaxation.

Combine melatonin pills with regular exercise and a healthy diet.

Before beginning anything, see a doctor. The key to optimum health is recognizing what your body requires.

Chapter 5:
Exercise and Practical Advice

Every stage of life benefits greatly from exercise. You'll feel younger, stronger, and more resistant to several ailments thanks to it.

A long process is required to lose weight. Sometimes our ideas about how to achieve our weight loss objectives prevent us from following through, leaving us discouraged and without success. You must adopt a new, healthy lifestyle that is straightforward to maintain if you want to lose weight and keep it off.

You can utilize the advice in the paragraphs below to lose weight and keep it off. There is no need to restrict certain foods, monitor calories, or starve yourself. The following strategy will help you lose weight steadily and eventually get to your target weight.

Great Guidance

Exercise will become much more important as you age, especially for weight loss and building muscle mass. Exercise will help you lose weight, but it will also help you keep it off in the long run. Recent research demonstrates that women who exercise regularly are more successful at controlling their weight than those who don't.

Aerobics is among the most beneficial exercises. While you burn calories, aerobic exercise will help you lose body fat from many places, including the area around your belly. It will also help you avoid the numerous health problems that it can bring.

You can work out at home a couple of days a week and achieve the same results as going to the gym. Don't expect a miracle to happen right away because it takes time. You can stop diseases linked to being overweight once you start doing aerobics.

Many people think that to maintain their health, they need to run 1 to 2 miles every day in addition to performing various other exercises. They frequently immediately stop exercising because of the notion. No matter how complicated or simple the action, fifteen to twenty minutes every day is advised. It will eventually pay off. A terrific fitness plan that can help you burn calories and move your entire body is brisk walking for twenty minutes.

Studies show that including aerobics in your daily routine and making it a physical activity, such as brisk daily walking, leaf raking, etc., is a well-structured exercise program that may improve heart activity, the respiratory system, and fitness, and will lower the risk of various diseases.

Additionally, you'll burn calories and body fat.

Now, if you increase your daily walking time to, say, a half-hour, you can develop a healthier lifestyle. You might go for a 15-minute walk in the morning and another 15-minute walk later in the day. Moving the muscles will bring you one step closer to a longer, healthier, and happier life.

You can burn calories by engaging in hobbies like housework, gardening, and other similar ones. Most people will put off till tomorrow what they might have done today. Try to avoid putting things off. Cleaning a tiny residence simply takes a few minutes, and once you're done, you'll enjoy the benefits.

Change your outlook. Delete your "goal weight." Instead of concentrating on how much weight you want to lose, use that same energy to focus on living a better lifestyle. Instead of focusing on how nice you appear on the exterior, concentrate on how good you seem on the "inside". When your internal organs are healthy, operating properly, and taken care of, you can lose weight for a long time.

Attempt to eat as "organically" as you can. The majority of prayers for weight loss are unanswered because of many of the meals that are consumed today. Conventional foods are laced with hormones, toxins, and pesticides that enter our bodies directly. If the beef you consume comes from a cow that was given hormone injections to help it grow bigger and quicker, it stands to reason that those hormones will also affect you.

Include a fruit or vegetable at every meal. Including fruits and veggies will help you feel fuller more quickly and provide you with vital nutrients that you don't typically get, even if you're eating something genuinely harmful.

Your body will "look great" both inside and out as a result.

Start eating more meals at home. The time required to drive, place an order, pick up, and bring meals home from a restaurant is at least 35 minutes. So why not prepare the same dish at home in those 35 minutes? It's healthier as you have more control over the ingredients and serving amounts, and you're less vulnerable to bacteria and other revolting things that weirdos do to people's food in public settings.

Get moving for at least 30 minutes every day, two of which should be low-impact. It's easy. Rather than driving, take a walk to the grocery shop. Spend a half-hour playing outside with your kids, or go dancing. Consider exercising as a necessity rather than a chore. The art of moving your body is all that it is! Make it a lifestyle choice. Find a physical activity schedule that you enjoy and follow it.

When you are hungry, eat. In the long run, failing to do so will only lead to overeating. Just be sure to control your portion sizes when you eat and occasionally "treat" yourself to something pleasant to prevent feelings of deprivation or punishment.

Do not eat if you are not hungry! Although it may seem like common sense, you wouldn't believe how often we practice it. We can easily "snack" even when we are not hungry. This behavior directly undermines your attempts to lose weight. Please stay away from it.

Keep a positive outlook on your physical appearance. Every time, stop yourself. Every time you think or speak negatively about your weight, eating habits, or body, stop yourself. If you stumble, immediately follow it up with a good idea or phrase. To achieve our objectives, we must accept the body we are in right now.

Conclusion

Your innate instincts were given to you at birth. Your gut feelings may be your best source of guidance. Consider this: Over the years, you may have heard that you may lose weight if you follow a certain eating plan. The majority of people live their lives trying to be someone they're not, thus no diet in the world will work for them.

Instincts may lead you to better health, but most people will ignore them. For instance, you were warned not to go to the pub last night. However, you might still go and then wonder why you don't feel good the next day.

You'll see the right way to choose if you let nature run its course. To get where you want to go, you must have intelligence.

Perception and intelligence are wisdom. When you use wisdom to make decisions, you exercise smart judgment and develop sharp ideas that enable you to see clearly. Knowledge advances common sense. By gaining information, comprehension, insight, and other skills, you can become wise. So begin right away.

One more thing...

Regardless of what you have experienced thus far in your effort to lose weight, think this is true right now.

Keeping your body satisfied will help you stop cravings. The easiest method to achieve this is to consume a protein-rich, wholesome breakfast in the morning to front-load your calories.

This will not only speed up your metabolism, causing your body to burn fat throughout the day, but it will also help you resist cravings that result in bad eating habits.

Having a healthy meal first thing in the morning not only speeds up your metabolism and keeps you burning calories all day long, but it also puts you in the right frame of mind to start the day strong as a "dieter"!

This is why breakfast is important. Your body is ready to go on the hunt for food when you first wake up in the morning. Your metabolism is in full swing, and your cortisol and adrenaline levels are at their highest.

Your brain signals your body to start looking for a different fuel source if you don't give it the energy it needs straight away.

As a result, it depletes the strength of your priceless and exquisite muscular tissue.

Even worse, your body and brain, which are still in starvation mode, will retain the energy you give them in the form of fat when you eat again later. Having a large, hearty breakfast, give your body exactly what it needs when it needs it, breaking the cycle of cravings that is so addictive.

Also, keep in mind:

1. Ideas are objects.

2. Words are strong.

3. Emotions and feelings provide the fuel and electricity needed to give your desires life.

4. Moving forward without first placing thoughts, words, and feelings in line before those actions gives actions greater force than doing so.

I hope this book has provided you with a solid foundation for your weight loss efforts.